Dummies type 2 diabetes guide 2023

The Ultimate Guide to Living a Healthy Life and Managing a Newly Diagnosed Type 2 Diabetes with a 30-Day Meal Plan and Easy, Sample Low-carb Recipes.

Dr. Stephen Campbell

Table of Contents

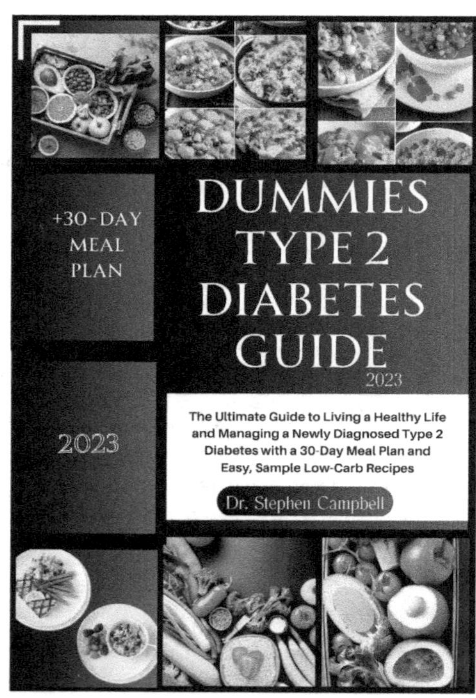

+30-DAY MEAL PLAN
2023
DUMMIES TYPE 2 DIABETES GUIDE
2023
The Ultimate Guide to Living a Healthy Life and Managing a Newly Diagnosed Type 2 Diabetes with a 30-Day Meal Plan and Easy, Sample Low-Carb Recipes
Dr. Stephen Campbell

Introduction

The past three years had been difficult for Lisa, a 42-year-old woman who had type 2 diabetes. She had experimented with a number of drugs and lifestyle modifications in an effort to manage her blood sugar, but nothing appeared to be working. She was starting to feel dejected and frustrated.

A book titled "Dummies type 2 diabetes guide" was discovered by Lisa one day while she was perusing a nearby bookstore. She chose to read it because she found the title intriguing.

The value of a healthy diet and regular exercise in controlling type 2 diabetes was covered in the book. The many accessible pharmaceutical types were also described, along with any possible side effects. The information captivated Lisa, who made the decision to test it out.

She began by altering her dietary habits and consuming more nutritious grains, fruits, and veggies. She started going to the gym frequently and making sure she got plenty of rest. After a few weeks, Lisa discovered to her joyful surprise that her blood sugar levels were improving.

Lisa proceeded to alter her way of life and food during the ensuing few months. Eventually, she succeeded in reversing her type 2 diabetes. She couldn't believe she could do this without taking any medication, and she was relieved.

Chapter 1

Understanding the Causes of Type 2 Diabetes

Millions of individuals worldwide suffer with type 2 diabetes, a chronic disease that is brought on by a combination of environmental, genetic, and lifestyle factors. High blood sugar levels are a defining feature of the illness, which can cause a number of major health issues.

You can lower your risk of getting type 2 diabetes by taking action by being aware of its causes.

Genetics

Diabetes type 2 is influenced by genetics. You might be more prone to developing the ailment if it runs in your family. According to research, people of particular races and ethnicities are more likely to develop type 2 diabetes.

Age

Your risk of type 2 diabetes may also be impacted by your age. Your risk increases as you age. Type 2 diabetes is more likely to strike adults over the age of 45 than it is younger ones.

Weight

Obesity and being overweight are significant risk factors for type 2 diabetes. The body's capacity to react to insulin, the hormone that aids in controlling blood sugar levels, can be lowered by obesity. Type 2 diabetes is more likely to strike overweight people than healthy-weight people.

Diet

You run a higher risk of developing type 2 diabetes if you consume a diet heavy in refined carbs, such as white bread and sugary beverages. Consuming excessive amounts of fried and processed food can also raise your risk.

Physical exercise

Another risk factor for type 2 diabetes is physical inactivity. Inactivity increases the likelihood of developing the illness compared to regular exercise.

Lifestyle

Your risk of type 2 diabetes may also rise if you smoke, consume alcohol, or sleep insufficiently. Stressed-out individuals may also be more prone to developing the illness.

You can lower your risk of getting type 2 diabetes by taking action after learning the causes of the disease. Your risk can be decreased by making lifestyle changes like eating a healthy diet, exercising frequently, and giving up smoking. A frequent health checkup might help you keep track of your risk of type 2 diabetes.

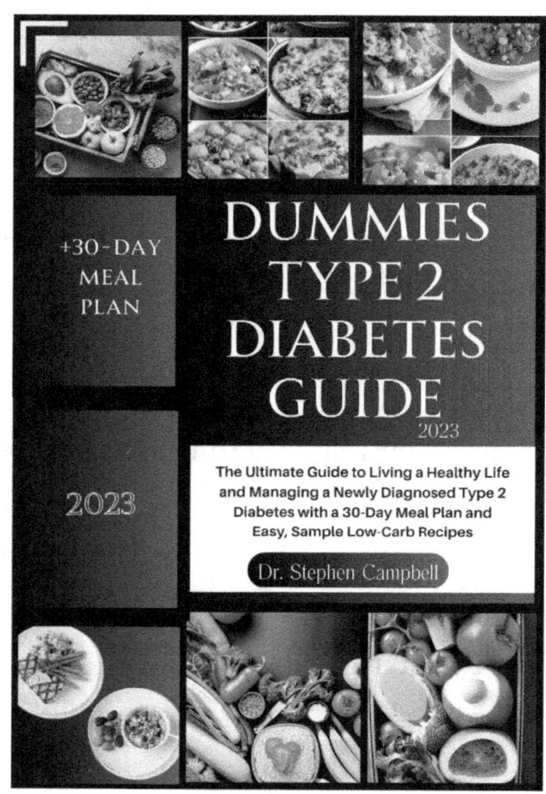

+30-DAY MEAL PLAN
2023
DUMMIES TYPE 2 DIABETES GUIDE
2023
The Ultimate Guide to Living a Healthy Life and Managing a Newly Diagnosed Type 2 Diabetes with a 30-Day Meal Plan and Easy, Sample Low-Carb Recipes
Dr. Stephen Campbell

Chapter 2

Managing Type 2 Diabetes

Following are some guidelines for controlling type 2 diabetes:

1. Regularly check your blood glucose levels. Doing this will enable you to see any changes in your levels and take the necessary action. A blood glucose meter can be used for this, or your doctor can check your levels on a regular basis.

2. Consume a nutritious diet: Maintaining a healthy diet is crucial for controlling type 2 diabetes. A balanced diet high in fiber, fruits, vegetables, and whole grains, low in sugar and saturated fat, and low in saturated fat and sugar can help you maintain stable blood sugar levels and avoid issues.

3. frequent exercise: Keeping your type 2 diabetes under control requires frequent exercise. Your body's sensitivity to insulin can be improved and blood glucose levels can be lowered with regular exercise. On most days of the week, try to get in at least 30 minutes of moderate exercise, such as walking, cycling, or swimming.

4. Take meds as directed: It's vital to follow your doctor's instructions if you've been given medication to manage type 2 diabetes. This can help you maintain appropriate blood sugar levels and avoid any problems.

5. Control your stress levels: Stress can increase blood sugar levels, therefore it's critical to control it to keep them within a healthy range. Exercises for reducing stress, such yoga, meditation, and mindfulness, can be beneficial.

6. Keep an eye on your feet: Diabetics are more prone to foot issues including infections and ulcers.

Regularly inspect your feet for any injury or infection symptoms, and get medical help if necessary.

7. Give up smoking: If you smoke, it's vital to stop because it might make type 2 diabetes symptoms worse. You can stop smoking with the aid of numerous tools, including counseling and nicotine replacement therapy.

By implementing these suggestions, type 2 diabetes can be managed and complications can be avoided. It is crucial to talk to your doctor if you have any queries or worries.

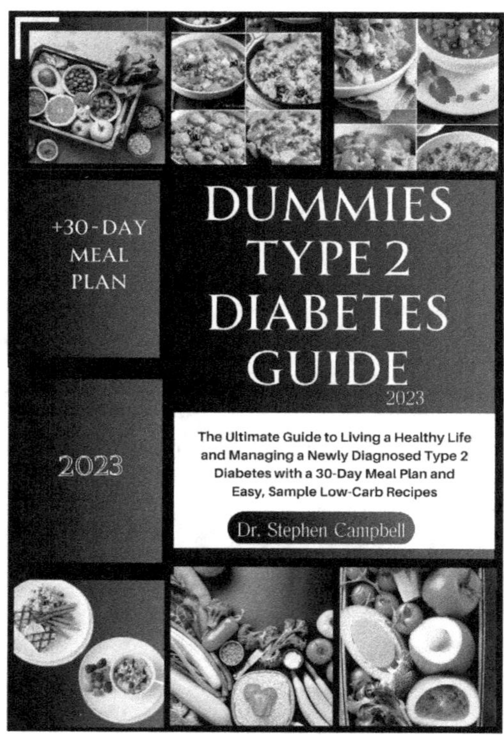

+30-DAY
MEAL
PLAN
2023
DUMMIES
TYPE 2
DIABETES
GUIDE
2023
The Ultimate Guide to Living a Healthy Life
and Managing a Newly Diagnosed Type 2
Diabetes with a 30-Day Meal Plan and
Easy, Sample Low-Carb Recipes
Dr. Stephen Campbell

Chapter 3

Diabetes Diet and Nutrition

Diet and nutrition for those with diabetes are crucial components of managing the disease and keeping one's health. Key elements of managing diabetes include eating a nutritious diet and controlling your macronutrient intake.

An appropriate ratio of carbs, proteins, and lipids should be included in a diabetes diet. Energy is provided by carbohydrates, proteins aid in the development and maintenance of biological tissues, and fats offer both energy and necessary fatty acids. For the best control of diabetes, eat a diversified diet rich in fruits, vegetables, whole grains, and lean meats.

Practice portion control and be sure to include foods that are high in vitamins and minerals in your diet in addition to maintaining a balanced diet. Maintaining blood sugar levels can be aided by eating regular meals and snacks throughout the day.

The following are 5 various forms of diabetic diets and nutrition:

1. Low-Carb Diet: This eating plan substitutes lean proteins and healthy fats for the carbohydrates that are often ingested.

2. Mediterranean Diet: This eating plan emphasizes consuming produce, whole grains, fish, and healthy fats that are often consumed in Mediterranean nations.

3. High Fiber Diet: This eating plan includes whole grains, legumes, fruits, and vegetables since they are high in fiber.

4. Low Glycemic Index Diet: This diet focuses on consuming foods with a low glycemic index, which means they are slowly digested and absorbed, helping to maintain stable blood sugar levels.

5. Ketogenic Diet: It has been shown that people with type 2 diabetes can benefit from this high-fat, low-carb diet.

There is no one-size-fits-all approach to diabetic diet and nutrition, and it is crucial to keep this in mind. Making sure that your specific requirements are met and that you are receiving the nutrition you require can be made easier by working with a licensed dietitian.

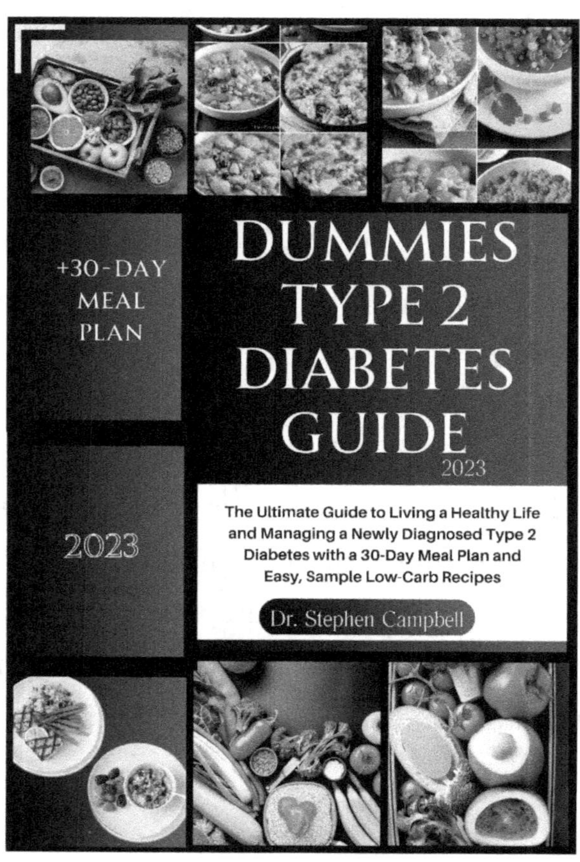
+30-DAY MEAL PLAN
2023
DUMMIES TYPE 2 DIABETES GUIDE
2023
The Ultimate Guide to Living a Healthy Life and Managing a Newly Diagnosed Type 2 Diabetes with a 30-Day Meal Plan and Easy, Sample Low-Carb Recipes
Dr. Stephen Campbell

Chapter 4

Exercise and Type 2 Diabetes

A crucial component of controlling Type 2 diabetes is exercise. You can regulate your blood sugar levels more effectively, decrease weight, and lower your risk of heart disease and stroke by engaging in regular physical activity. Additionally, exercise can strengthen your bones and muscles, improve your circulation, and increase your mood and energy.

Consider the following exercise categories:

Exercises that are aerobic include jogging, swimming, biking, hiking, and walking.

• Resistance training: Strengthening and muscle-building exercises of this kind. Examples include lifting weights, utilizing resistance bands, or performing exercises like pushups and squats using only your body weight.

Exercises for flexibility and stretching can help you increase your range of motion and lessen stiffness. Pilates, yoga, and tai chi are a few examples.

• Balance drills: These drills help you become more coordinated and stable. Examples include doing heel lifts, walking heel to toe, and standing on one leg.

Regardless of the workout you select, it's crucial to see your doctor before beginning a new fitness regimen. They can assist you in developing a plan that is suitable for your needs, safe, and effective. Additionally, it's crucial to hydrate well and warm up and cool down before and after each exercise session.

Regular exercise can significantly improve your health and assist you in controlling your diabetes.

Therefore, if you're searching for a way to enhance your general health, think about including physical activity in your daily schedule.

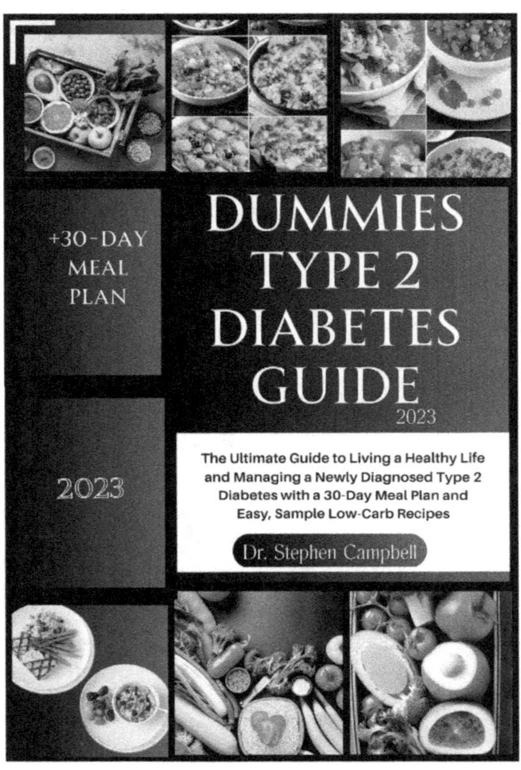

+30-DAY
MEAL
PLAN

2023

DUMMIES
TYPE 2
DIABETES
GUIDE
2023

The Ultimate Guide to Living a Healthy Life
and Managing a Newly Diagnosed Type 2
Diabetes with a 30-Day Meal Plan and
Easy, Sample Low-Carb Recipes

Dr. Stephen Campbell

Chapter 5

Medications and Treatments

A chronic illness, type 2 diabetes can be controlled through dietary adjustments, medication, and other therapies. Maintaining blood glucose levels within a specific range is the main objective of treatment to lower the risk of problems.

An essential component of type 2 diabetes management is medication. It is used to lower the risk of problems and help keep blood glucose levels within the desired range. It is possible to utilize insulin, sulfonylureas, meglitinides, thiazolidinediones, dipeptidyl peptidase-4 inhibitors, and glucagon-like peptide-1 agonists among other types of medication. Every medicine has a unique mechanism of action and a unique set of potential adverse effects.

Changes in lifestyle are also crucial for managing type 2 diabetes. Stress reduction, a nutritious diet, and regular exercise can all help keep blood sugar levels within the desired range. It's crucial to stop smoking because it raises your chance of problems.

Type 2 diabetes can be managed with additional therapies. These include undergoing weight loss surgery, using an insulin pump, and continuously monitoring glucose levels.

To properly control type 2 diabetes, it may occasionally be required to use a mix of prescription drugs, lifestyle modifications, and other treatments. The ideal treatment strategy for your particular needs should be determined in collaboration with a healthcare professional.

Chapter 6

Living Well with Type 2 Diabetes

With the appropriate attitude and lifestyle, living well with Type 2 Diabetes is feasible. Chronic Type 2 Diabetes alters how your body metabolizes blood sugar, which results in elevated blood sugar levels. Although there is no cure for this condition, it can be managed with the right care.

The first step in delaying or preventing the onset of Type 2 Diabetes is to take preventive measures. This entails getting regular exercise, following a healthy diet, keeping a healthy weight, and limiting or abstaining from alcohol and tobacco use.

Second, it's crucial to periodically check your blood sugar levels. You can check your blood sugar levels at home using a glucose meter or by going to the doctor for routine blood sugar checks.

Thirdly, it's crucial to take your prescriptions exactly as your physician has instructed. This includes drugs that lower blood sugar levels and drugs that lessen your chance of developing disease-related problems.

Fourth, it's crucial to adopt a healthy lifestyle. This entails maintaining a regular exercise schedule and eating a balanced diet low in salt, sugar, and fat. Get proper rest and manage your stress as well.

For support and direction, it's crucial to keep in touch with your doctor and other medical experts. They can assist you in modifying your lifestyle to maintain healthy blood sugar levels.

With the correct attitude, a change in lifestyle, and support, living well with Type 2 Diabetes is feasible. You can control your diabetes and live a healthy, meaningful life with help and dedication.

Chapter 7

30 days meal plan and preparation

Day 1:

Breakfast consists of oatmeal with almond milk and fresh fruit.

Lunch will be a salad with grilled chicken, mixed greens, tomatoes, cucumbers, and olive oil vinaigrette.

Fruit and cottage cheese for a snack

Dinner will be roasted veggies and baked salmon.

Day 2:

Breakfast consists of whole-wheat bread with banana and peanut butter.

Lunch will be a baked sweet potato with salsa and black beans.

Greek yogurt, chopped nuts, and dried fruit for a snack

Dinner will be grilled shrimp and stir-fried vegetables.

Day 3:
Eggs scrambled with bell peppers and mushrooms for breakfast

Quinoa and black bean tortilla for lunch

Snack: Hummus-topped celery sticks.

Dinner will be vegan chili.

Day 4:

Greek yogurt and fruit smoothie for breakfast.

Lunchtime sandwich of turkey, lettuce, tomato, and avocado

Apple slices with peanut butter as a snack

Roasted chicken and broccoli for dinner

Day 5:

Breakfast: Chia-seed-infused overnight oats.

Tzatziki and baked falafel for lunch

Snack: Hummus and carrot sticks.

Lenten soup for supper

Day 6:

Egg-white omelet with bell peppers and spinach for breakfast

Salad of grilled salmon, mixed greens, tomatoes, and balsamic vinaigrette for lunch.

Almond butter on celery sticks as a snack

Dinner will be baked sweet potatoes with salsa and black beans.

Day 7:
Breakfast includes avocado on whole wheat toast.

Quinoa and veggie stir-fry for lunch.

Greek yogurt and granola for a snack

Dinner will be grilled shrimp and a green salad.

Day 8:
Oatmeal with berries and almonds for breakfast

Tzatziki and baked falafel for lunch

Apple slices with peanut butter as a snack

Eggplant Parmesan for supper

Day 9:
Greek yogurt and fruit smoothie for breakfast.

Lunch will be a salad of grilled chicken, mixed greens, tomatoes, and olive oil vinaigrette.

Snack: Hummus and carrot sticks.

Lenten soup for supper

Day 10:
Eggs scrambled with bell peppers and mushrooms for breakfast

Quinoa and black bean tortilla for lunch

Almond butter on celery sticks as a snack

Dinner will be roasted veggies and baked salmon.

Day 11:
Breakfast consists of whole-wheat bread with banana and peanut butter.

Salad of grilled salmon, mixed greens, tomatoes, and balsamic vinaigrette for lunch.

Greek yogurt, chopped nuts, and dried fruit for a snack

Dinner will be vegan chili.

Day 12:
Breakfast: Chia-seed-infused overnight oats.

Lunchtime sandwich of turkey, lettuce, tomato, and avocado

Fruit and cottage cheese for a snack

Roasted chicken and broccoli for dinner

Day 13:
Egg-white omelet with bell peppers and spinach for breakfast

Lunch will be a baked sweet potato with salsa and black beans.

Snack: Hummus-topped celery sticks.

Dinner will be grilled shrimp and stir-fried vegetables.

Day 14:
Breakfast consists of oatmeal with almond milk and fresh fruit.

Quinoa and veggie stir-fry for lunch.

Apple slices with peanut butter as a snack

Eggplant Parmesan for supper

Day 15:
Greek yogurt and fruit smoothie for breakfast.

Lunch will be a salad with grilled chicken, mixed greens, tomatoes, cucumbers, and olive oil vinaigrette.

Snack: Hummus and carrot sticks.

Lenten soup for supper

Day 16:
Breakfast includes avocado on whole wheat toast.

Tzatziki and baked falafel for lunch

Almond butter on celery sticks as a snack

Dinner will be roasted veggies and baked salmon.

Day 17:

Eggs scrambled with bell peppers and mushrooms for breakfast

Quinoa and black bean tortilla for lunch

Greek yogurt and granola for a snack

Dinner will be vegan chili.

Day 18:

Breakfast: Chia-seed-infused overnight oats.

Salad of grilled salmon, mixed greens, tomatoes, and balsamic vinaigrette for lunch.

Fruit and cottage cheese for a snack

Roasted chicken and broccoli for dinner

Day 19:

Breakfast consists of whole-wheat bread with banana and peanut butter.

Lunch will be a baked sweet potato with salsa and black beans.

Apple slices with peanut butter as a snack

Dinner will be grilled shrimp and a green salad.

Day 20:
Egg-white omelet with bell peppers and spinach for breakfast

Lunchtime sandwich of turkey, lettuce, tomato, and avocado

Snack: Hummus-topped celery sticks.

Eggplant Parmesan for supper

Day 21:

Oatmeal with berries and almonds for breakfast

Quinoa and veggie stir-fry for lunch.

Snack: Hummus and carrot sticks.

Lenten soup for supper

Day 22:

Greek yogurt and fruit smoothie for breakfast.

Lunch will be a salad of grilled chicken, mixed greens, tomatoes, and olive oil vinaigrette.

Greek yogurt, chopped nuts, and dried fruit for a snack

Dinner will be roasted veggies and baked salmon.

Day 23:

Breakfast includes avocado on whole wheat toast.

Tzatziki and baked falafel for lunch

Almond butter on celery sticks as a snack

Dinner will be vegan chili.

Day 24:
Eggs scrambled with bell peppers and mushrooms
for breakfast

Salad of grilled salmon, mixed greens, tomatoes,
and balsamic vinaigrette for lunch.

Fruit and cottage cheese for a snack

Roasted chicken and broccoli for dinner

Day 25:
Breakfast: Chia-seed-infused overnight oats.

Quinoa and black bean tortilla for lunch

Apple slices with peanut butter as a snack

Dinner will be grilled shrimp and stir-fried vegetables.

Day 26:
Breakfast consists of oatmeal with almond milk and fresh fruit.

Lunch will be a baked sweet potato with salsa and black beans.

Snack: Hummus and carrot sticks.

Eggplant Parmesan for supper

Day 27:
Breakfast consists of whole-wheat bread with banana and peanut butter.

Lunch will be a salad with grilled chicken, mixed greens, tomatoes, cucumbers, and olive oil vinaigrette.

Almond butter on celery sticks as a snack

Lenten soup for supper

Day 28:
Egg-white omelet with bell peppers and spinach for breakfast

Tzatziki and baked falafel for lunch

Greek yogurt and granola for a snack

Dinner will be roasted veggies and baked salmon.

Day 29:

Greek yogurt and fruit smoothie for breakfast.

Quinoa and veggie stir-fry for lunch.

Snack: Hummus-topped celery sticks.

Dinner will be vegan chili.

Day 30:
Breakfast: Chia-seed-infused overnight oats.

Lunchtime sandwich of turkey, lettuce, tomato, and avocado

Apple slices with peanut butter as a snack

Roasted chicken and broccoli for dinner

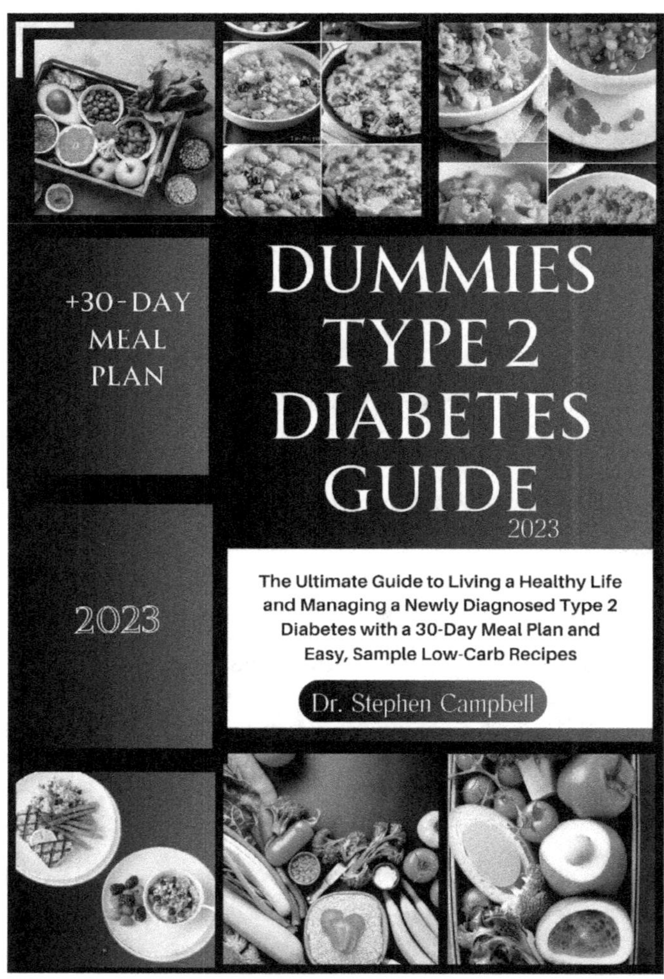

+30-DAY MEAL PLAN
2023
DUMMIES TYPE 2 DIABETES GUIDE
2023
The Ultimate Guide to Living a Healthy Life and Managing a Newly Diagnosed Type 2 Diabetes with a 30-Day Meal Plan and Easy, Sample Low-Carb Recipes
Dr. Stephen Campbell

9 7 9 8 3 9 3 8 1 0 0 0 9